# Health Benefits of Meditation

## by M. Usman

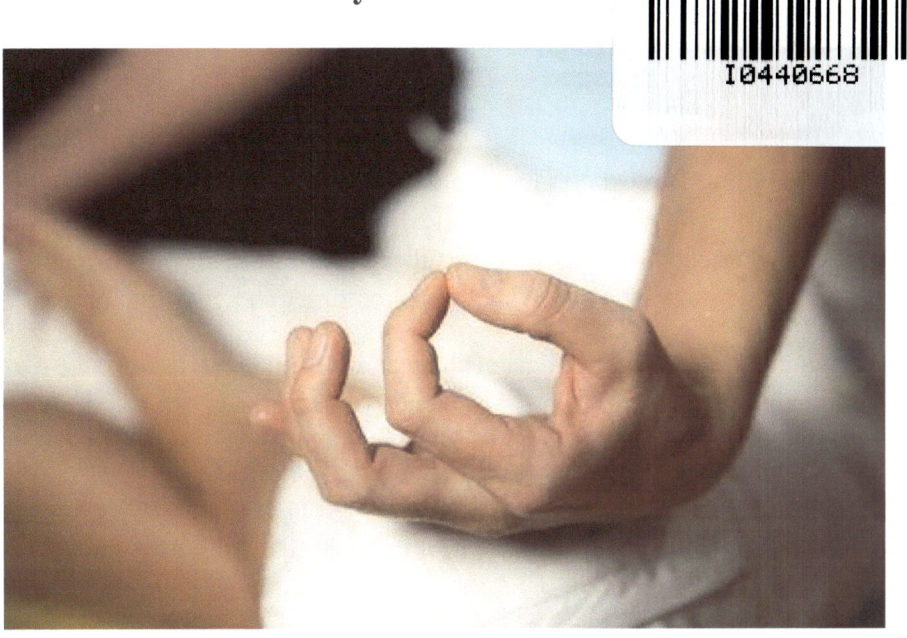

**Health Learning Series**

**Mendon Cottage Books**

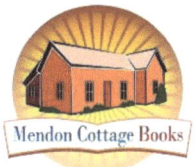

*JD-Biz Publishing*

**Disclaimer**

The information is this book is provided for informational purposes only. It is not intended to be used and medical advice or a substitute for proper medical treatment by a qualified health care provider. The information is believed to be accurate as presented based on research by the author.

The contents have not been evaluated by the U.S. Food and Drug Administration or any other Government or Health Organization and the contents in this book are not to be used to treat cure or prevent disease.

The author or publisher are not responsible for the use or safety of any diet, procedure or treatment mentioned in this book. The author or publisher is not responsible for errors or omissions that may exist.

**Warning**

The Book is for informational purposes only and before taking on any diet, treatment or medical procedure it is recommended to consult with your primary care provider.

## Our books are available at

1. Amazon.com

2. Barnes and Noble

3. Itunes

4. Kobo

5. Smashwords

6. Google Play Books

# Table of Contents

# Preface

Social pressure, packed schedules and flailing economies; who has time or the money to even think, let alone practice any type of fitness or health regime. Even those who have the gift of time soon find themselves stuck in the web of, what is mostly an artificial and synthetic dieting market, not realizing they would totally be at the mercy of the industry that's just out there for their money.

In this deranged scene, a world wide revival was made by an art, practiced for over a thousands of years, 'meditation'. Shooting to fame in the 60s, meditation has been the subject of thousands of scientific studies, with the most heavy ones being taken after the 70s. What is meditation? When most people listen to the word meditation, the image of a Buddhist monk sitting in a weird position comes to mind. This, no doubt is the main idea behind meditation, is still not the extent of it. Before knowing what meditation is, you must know what it is not.

Meditation is not:

- **Concentration:** An attempt to hold one's attention on one specific idea or entity for a usually, long period of time. The techniques used in meditation are just a bit related to the word.

- **Losing Control:** Voices, sounds, involuntary movements and spasms have no relation with meditation. These are just signs of loss of awareness, showing that one no longer controls some or most of his/her body.

- **Exercises:** Physical positions, postures and heavy breathing are also not meditation. These practices can help establish a greater balance in your body, but only if practiced under the supervision of a master. Without a master's guidance, you'll just be hindering your body's to channel its energy in the right way.

- **Mental effort:** For instance, if you keep on thinking about one thing you won't go anywhere with your practice.

Meditation is a tool that helps you rediscover your own inner intelligence. It is keeping the mind quiet, finding the silence that already runs in our nerves and making it an active part of the life. From this increased sense of awareness, you attain intuition, inspiration and complete control and connection, down to the last nerve of the body. In effect you gain countless benefits, not just emotional or spiritual but physical too; you block out countless allergies, disorders and diseases that can or have ravaged through your body. Remember that there is no one way to meditate and in comparison one way is not better than the other as they all use the same principle at the core.

In this book you'll learn all about the benefits of meditation, how it is done and how it provides relief by using only the body's own ability and not any medication. You will see that nature doesn't put a cost on health and well-being.

So forget about your stress and take and relax, because your life is about to get a lot better!

# Getting Started

## Chapter # 1: Intro

Originally meditation was a mean to attain an in-depth knowledge of the mystical and spiritual forces present in nature. However, these days the scene has pretty much changed and meditation has become a way for relaxing and reducing stress.

Meditation is neither a diet nor a fitness regime. Meditation is an effortless practice rendering a state that neutralizes stress producing activity of the brain without causing any negative effects to the effectiveness and alertness to the brain; it is more of a medicine, hidden inside you, a mind-body harmonizing one that incurs a streamlined state of relaxation and a serene mind. During this state you eliminate every disturbing thought worrying your mind, causing stress or troubling you. This procedure invokes a well-balanced and enhanced emotional and physical state in your body.

# Chapter # 2: Why Meditate?

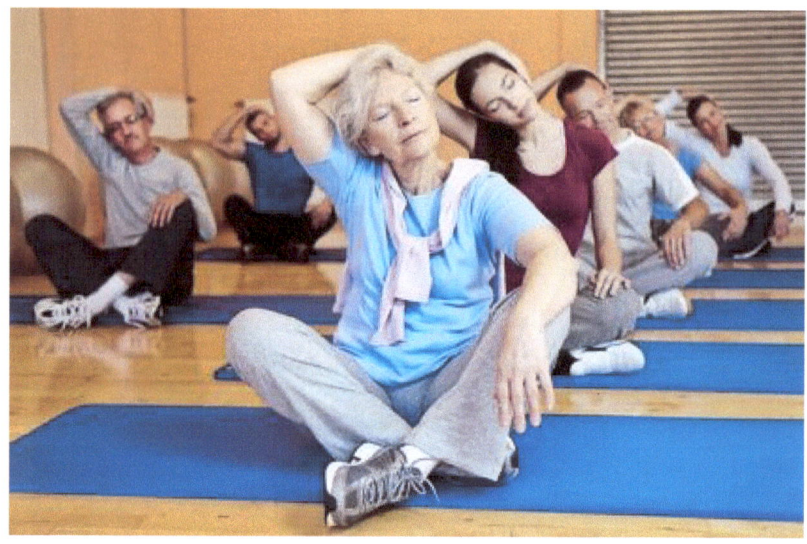

Anyone can reap the benefits of meditation. There are numerous reasons as to why you should switch to meditation, the first one being the simplicity and inexpensiveness. Meditation does not require you to buy special equipment or any kind of personalized meals for it to work. It doesn't even require a trainer or a gym. That's right you can practice meditation wherever you want, whenever you want; whether you're out on a walk, on the bus or giving an important as well as difficult presentation. If stress has resorted you to nail biting, consider meditation. Only a few moments of it will make you calm and relieve control of your nerves.

A study carried out by the US Medical Association in a time frame of six months showed that patients who underwent short courses of behavior modification strategies; i.e. meditation, went to their physicians significantly less than those who didn't. The savings made by employing this method were estimated at over 200 US Dollars per patient! Putting aside the physical and spiritual help that meditation does, meditation has a huge monetary benefit too as it increases the quality of one's life by reducing medical care bills; money that can be well spent on other stuff.

The following are the spiritual benefits one gains from meditation:

- Getting a new perspective, when in stressful situations.

- Development of a skill that helps in stress management.

- A higher conscious or self-awareness.

- Switching focus from the past or future to the present.

- Rooting out negative emotions and filling the space with positive ones.

The effects of meditation are not limited to mental well-being; meditation is also very useful to those with medical conditions, especially those that get stronger by stress. A growing number of researchers are concluding their researches to the point that meditation's ability of stress reduction inevitably benefits the whole body.

The conditions that alleviate through the practice of meditation include and are not limited to:

- Cancer

- Asthma

- Allergies

- Fatigue

- High Blood Pressure

- Anxiety disorders

- Binge eating

- Depression

- Heart disease

- Pain in joints

- Sleep problems

- Substance Abuse

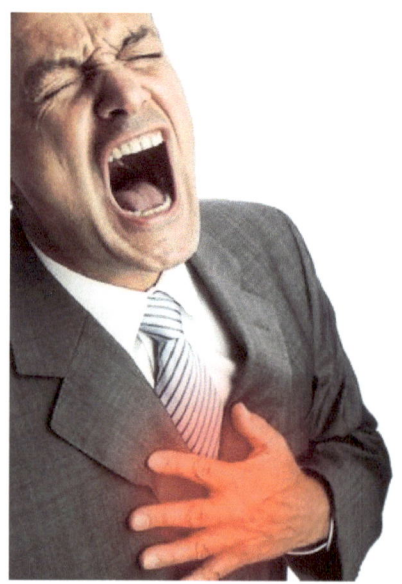

There is one thing that is highly recommended before you start practicing meditation; i.e. consult your doctor as there are some health conditions that can worsen with meditation rather than going the other way.

# Chapter # 3: Types of Meditation

The wait is over and the time has arrived for you to know how to practice meditation. Have you tried meditating before but ended up thinking it wasn't made for you? Numerous people ardently believe in meditation and the ways in which it helps the body strengthen it, but have a lot of difficulty practicing the art of meditation. Many people don't even know the numerous methods of meditation and usually end up doing the most common lotus position.

Below are some types of meditation discussed in detail that will definitely open your mind up to the world of meditation.

**Walking Meditation:**

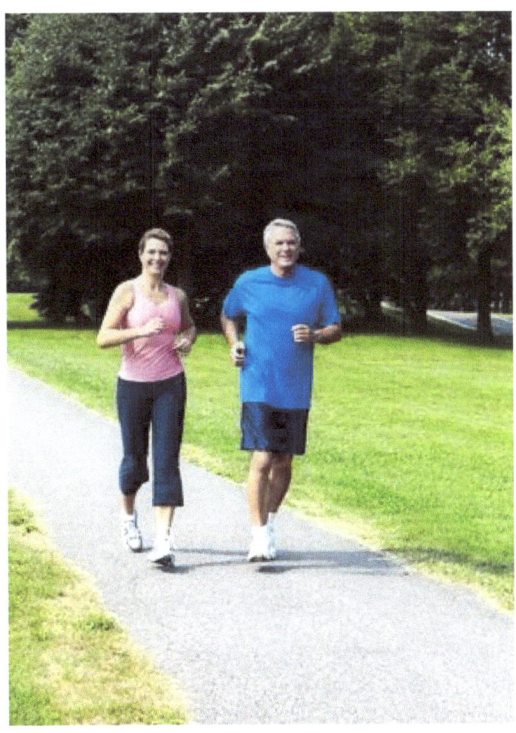

That's right! You can meditate even while you're walking. The biggest problem beginner face is sitting down for a long period of time therefore; walking meditation is the best choice for them. Walking meditation is just as good as sitting meditation. In addition it has the benefit of merging meditative experience into our daily life activities; it allows you to be present in your body and live in the moment.

It is best to perform this technique outdoors. Set aside 20 minutes for meditation and don't combine it with other stuff like errands or exercise.

Before walking, stand up and spend a little time getting aware of your body while staying still. Take a deep breath, right into the belly and pay full attention on the whole sensation while you breathe. Return your breathing pattern back to normal and notice while your body takes over. Now turn your attention back to your body; try to notice the feelings running through your body. Start walking in a relaxed and fairly normal state of mind. Naturally, your attention would be diverted to your surroundings so try your best to focus on what's going on inside you.

The general idea is to be attentive to the physical experience of walking. Your mind will wander off eventually so just imagine how your feet make alterations and your arms sway from left to right to keep your focus. Notice how your soles feel as they make contact with the socks, grass or sand as you walk. Feel the entire foot as one part of the foot makes contact with the ground. Gradually, shift your attention to other parts and joints of the body, like; ankles, calves, knees, etc. Feel all the tension that sits in these places and let it go. Then shift your attention to another part of the body and repeat. It is best to 'scan' your body for tension in a bottom-up method as it is more manageable but there is no restriction if you want to mix things up!

## Breath Awareness Meditation:

This technique falls in the sitting category of meditation.

Sit upright keeping your spine as straight as possible; straighten it to an extent at which you feel comfortable and don't force anything on your body as it is important for your body to relax completely. Now close your eyes and take a few moments to notice what's around you; the sounds, thoughts, feelings. Just notice them and don't try to alter them in any way. Do this while at the same time settle down.

After settling down in your surroundings shift your focus to the pattern of your breathing. Just feel how your breath moves in and moves out as the body automatically performs the inhaling and exhaling. Don't manipulate or change the breathing pattern in any way, let your body do its thing.

You'll soon find your mind wandering off into other places, away from breath so don't worry as it's all a part of it. As soon as this happens take a deep breath to bring the mind's attention where it must be. Let all your emotions, feelings and sensations float through your body as you focus on breathing. Notice how these sensations come and go in the same pattern as you inhale and exhale.

Soon, you will become aware of every bad feeling in your mind and you'll see how certain feelings are easy to let go compared to others. The natural relaxation state will help you cleanse your mind of every negative effect holding you back and disturbing you. Let it out of your body as you breathe out; try to think of a strong breeze that pulls it away and fill that part of your memory with something good and blissful. If you think you're having too much of a trouble letting a few memories go then leave it and don't apply any force as it won't help. Bring your attention back to this feeling when one cleansing cycle completes.

20 Minutes is the minimum time frame for this meditative technique.

**Basic Nature Meditation:**

As the name suggests, nature meditations are performed in a natural environment. Nature meditation enhances the core intelligence of nature in your physiology. Every part of our body responds to every little detail in nature such as the sound of a bird, smell of mud and the sensation of a breeze. Many people are already familiar with this phenomenon without even studying meditation!

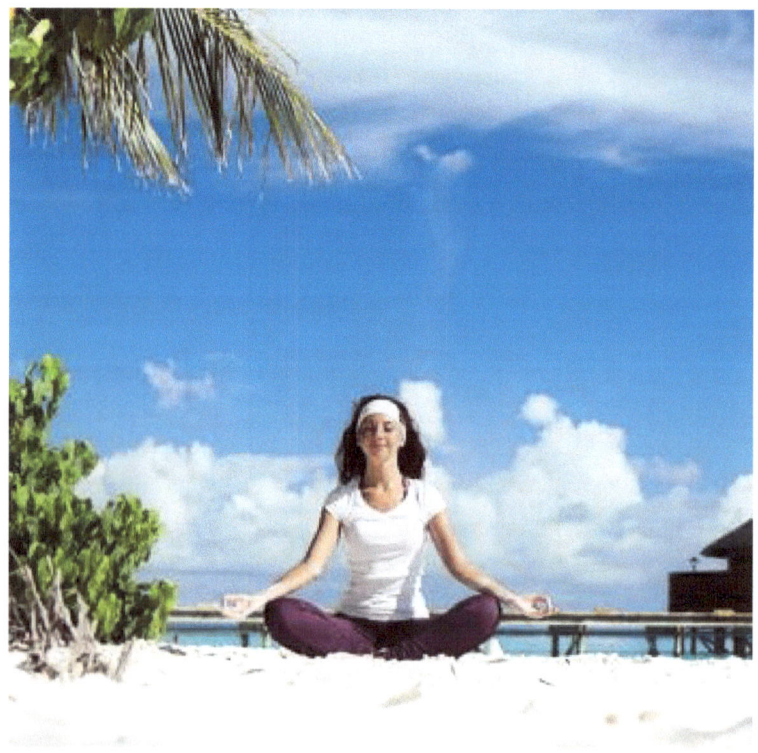

During this practice you are required to focus on the experience of nature using your senses with the exception of sight as your eyes would be closed during the process. So find a comfortable place in your garden or a nearby park and sit down in whichever position that suits you. Before closing your eyes take a few deep breaths deep into the belly. This will help you relax and prepare for the meditation. Now close your eyes and let your body take over the breathing; experience everything in nature with your eyes closed. Take note of how your whole body and mind feel. Experience the emotions running in your body without trying to alter them in any way. Keep doing this for about a minute or two and then shift your whole focus to your surroundings and what you feel as a consequence of it. For instance feel the air as it passes across your skin, feel the heat of the sun, listen to the cricketing, chirping sound of bees and birds respectively. During the rest of the meditative process keep focusing on these sensations. Don't panic as your mind wanders and gently bring it back on the nature rail.

During meditation, you will notice that your attention will be drawn to specific thoughts and experiences. Many of these will be good ones while some may be bad. For example a bird chirping may remind you of a similar song or sound you heard earlier. You might have heard the sound in the background while something terrible was going on and thus, the thought will immediately come to your mind. Focus on that thought and try to dissolve it within the chirping and get it out of your mind without applying to much force. Try this method to scan every different thought that comes up in your mind and treat it in the way it suits you; highlight the good effects and try to outweigh the bad ones with the positive energy that builds up as you cleanse your thoughts.

The time frame is same as before: 20 minutes at least.

# Chapter # 4: General Guidelines to Meditation

Here are some basic guidelines that will definitely help you clear up many of the confusions you have about meditation.

## Posture:

There are numerous postures for meditation and they all have different effect on how energy flows in your body. For most meditations sitting would be the optimum choice; sit in an upright position with the spine erect to a level that is comfortable to you. Notice that the last part of the previous sentence is of importance as you will not be able to completely relax if you're muscles or joints are strained.

## Length of time for meditation:

For starters 5 to 10 minutes of meditation is good but as you progress it's best to take your practice between 15 – 30 minutes. Start meditating from 5 minutes and gradually add five more minutes each subsequent week.

## When to meditate:

You can meditate at any time you wish however the recommended time is early in the morning to boost your day or in the afternoon when you want to unwind after a tough day at work.

Meditation will best help you relax when performed with an empty stomach or a few hours after a meal at the minimum.

## Meditation frequencies:

Once or twice a day is the ideal frequency for meditation. This combined with a regular routine is invaluable to your body and mind. You will benefit more if you meditate regularly rather than meditating on odd days or some other pattern. Remember that if you meditate more than twice a day could turn out to be counter-productive so just keep it balanced.

## Thought process:

As we let our mind settle down during meditation, the brain automatically triggers into a deeper level of thinking. Thoughts may turn into feelings that are hard to explain in mere words. Do not stop this process and let it take over you. Sometimes you may find yourself in a semi-dream kind of situation, being asleep and awake; this is a natural phenomenon and with practice can lead to the state of 'no thought' that every meditation practitioner wants to achieve.

## Noise:

Everyone wants to meditate in a quiet, nice corner but unfortunately it is not always possible. Each of the meditation techniques mentioned above can be practiced in noise as well; there's just one little secret and that is not to resist noise or force block it. Just let it be there and carry on. Go with the flow of things rather than against it and soon your mind will automatically negate these sounds for you.

## Falling asleep during meditation:

The true goal of every meditative technique is to help you achieve the state of 'non-resistance'; sleep will not be resisted by the mind as it comes and if an attempt is made to resist intentionally you will end up straining yourself. If you find that you fall asleep too often during meditation, the only plausible explanation is lack of sleep at night. Even though, there's no harm in sleeping while meditation; you can stop it by increasing your sleeping hours.

## Initiating the end of the meditative process:

Take your time to come out of the relaxed state you are in during meditation. Any haste in breaking the deep, meditative cycle can adversely affect your mind as well as your body. Keep your eyes closed for a minute and start moving your hands and arms for the purpose of stretching them. Finally, open your eyes and get up slowly. Walk a few steps and do whatever you want then!

# Benefits of Meditation to the Brain

## Chapter # 5: Behind the scenes

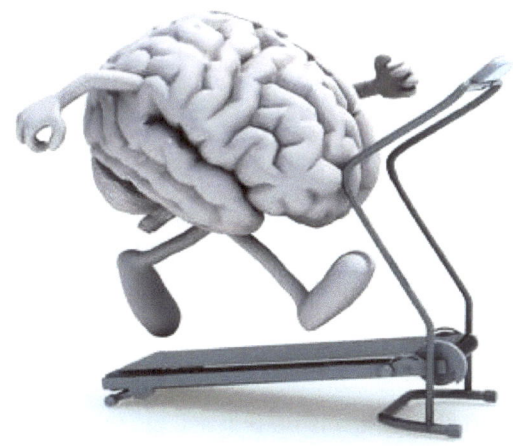

This is the part where things get simplified; Thanks to the modern technology like Real-time Magnetic Resonance Imaging, researchers have shown how meditation helps to improve our body. Scans of one's brain can reveal a lot about meditation. In simple words, the brain is made to slow the flow and processing of information as compared to the normal rate. The evidence for this comes from the sudden drop in flow of beta rays. Beta rays are an indication of processing in the brain; during meditation a decrease in the flow is noticed. A little more detailed is provided below.

The brain can be divided into three parts in context to meditation; the frontal lobe, the parietal lobe, and the thalamus. Don't get scared of the names as they're just for future references.

- The frontal lobe is the most complex part; it is responsible for logic, planning and emotions. Meditation tends to turn off this part.

- The parietal lobe is responsible for processing data we gain from our five senses. The activity in this part slows down during meditation.

- The thalamus is responsible for filtering sensory data; it only allows the important stuff pass through it. Meditation reduces this flow of information dramatically.

This slowdown results in a decrease in the load on the nerves and neurons and therefore, a chain reaction sets up that affects the whole body positively.

# Chapter # 6: Better focus & Greater Emotional Response

Focusing is a vital pillar of meditation. During meditation you practice to prevent your attention from falling into the wrong places; therefore, meditation improves focus during the non-meditative state. The result is quite simple. If you're a teenager, better grades; if you're a businessman, better presentations. In general it improves the quality of your work as well as personal life.

Research has also shown that people who meditate have an improved emotional response. Study conducted by *Emotion* magazine showed that people who meditate showed more sympathy towards disturbing content compared to people who don't meditate. This behavior was supported by a real time MRI of the amygdala – the part of the brain that controls emotional stimuli. This part of the brain responded exceptionally well with the meditative group. Therefore, meditation can be used to convert a cold blooded marine into a fitting member of the society!

# Chapter # 7: More Creativity and Better memory

Creativity is a make or break rule for writers. In fact every job nowadays requires you to take imitative and risks. Researchers of Leiden University studied the effects of meditation on creative skills. Those who did not practice meditation showed no change in their creativity and imagination towards a creativity task while those who did were filled with colorful ideas.

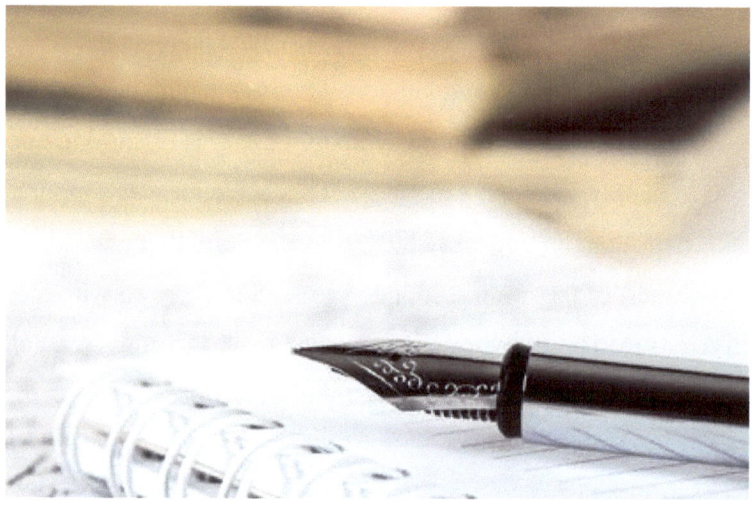

Everybody wants and loves to have a responsive memory. A lot of people diagnose themselves with Alzheimer disease when they fail to recall a name of a song or an actor. In fact the brain is so clogged up and distorted that at times it fails to make the right connections. Researchers at Martinos Center for Bio-Medical Imaging showed that practitioners of meditation were able to respond much rapidly to a memory test as compared those who did not meditate. They were able to ignore their distractions and had a much superior ability to recall facts.

# Chapter # 8: Less Stress& Anxiety

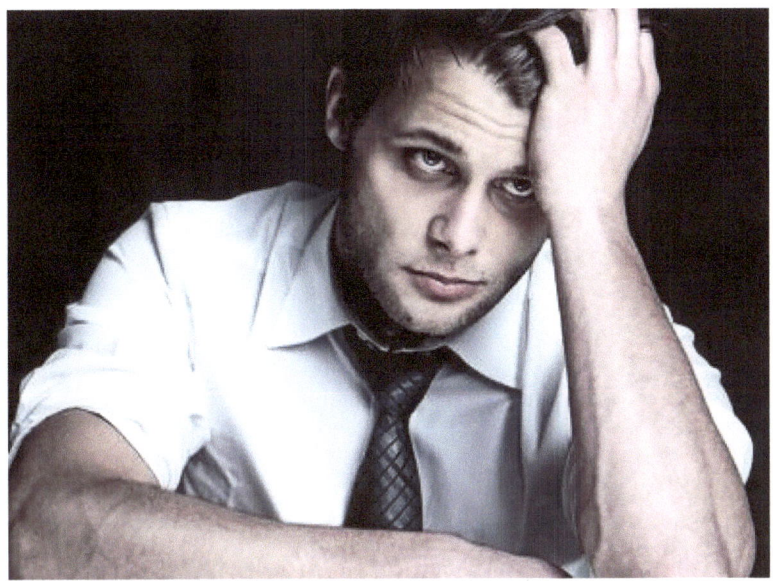

Stress is a benefit everyone knows and associates with meditation. It is the main culprit behind a ton of diseases and is the main target of meditation. A private study conducted in 2012 targeted human resource managers by dividing them into three separate groups. One group was given meditative training; the second was given body relaxation training while the third was given no training at all. After the eight week training program a grueling, stressful test was given to each of the groups within a time limit. The meditative group was able to perform most efficiently in the tests than both of the other groups.

Meditation helps manage anxiety better by loosening some of the connections in the brain. Don't worry; it's not bad at all! There is a part of the brain called medial prefrontal cortex that deals with personal information such as our experiences. Everyone carries bad memories and this is exactly the part where meditation comes in. Meditation weakens the neural connections that make you feel scared or under attack. In addition to loosening these connections meditation strengthens the connections in the reasoning part of the brain so you look at the matter with more logic than emotion.

# Benefits of Meditation to the Body

## Chapter # 9: Better Immunity

Your immunity system is your last line of defense against viruses and bacteria. It is a complex biological structure and if it gets weak it adversely affects the body's health. Meditation has proven itself a holistic way to strengthen the immune system.

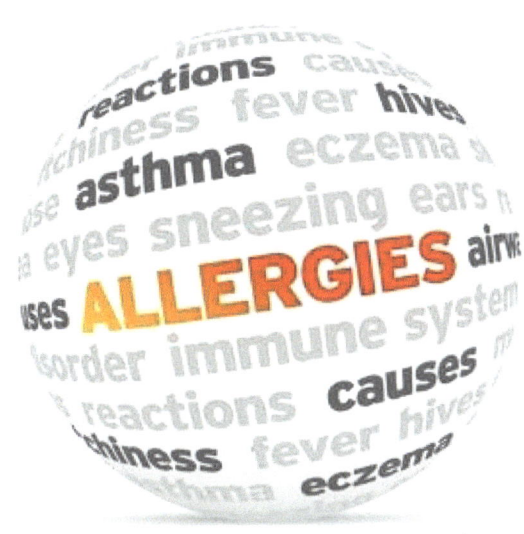

The immune system acts like a bridge between the mind and the body. It is affected by both negative and positive thoughts but at the same time is a biological structure. Improvement of the condition of one's brain directly affects the immune system's ability to cope with an attack. It's a common clinical observation that individuals exposed to stressful stimulus, depression and anxiety are more prone to develop diseases and infections.

What meditation has to do with immune system? You might ask. The answer is quite simple. As meditation alleviates stress and removes negative thoughts from the mind, as a result the body experiences a better flow of oxygen and blood. Meditative practices increase the amount of antibodies and as mentioned in the previous section enhances brain function; both of these factors contribute to the fortification of the immunity system. Meditation increases the activity in the left side of the brain that manages the immune system; as a result the immune system acts faster and more defensive cells are produced.

# Chapter # 10: Control on Blood Pressure

This is a fact that has been approved and recognized by hundreds of physicians across the globe. Multi-billion dollar drug companies have even carried out researches to prove it wrong but they have failed terribly.

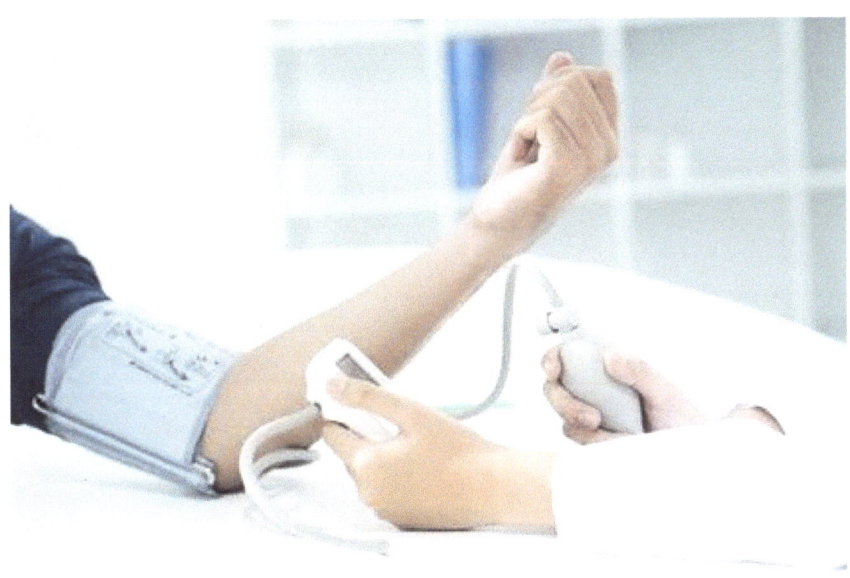

Meditation combined with a natural diet can do wonders for the body in terms of leveling blood to optimum pressure. Stress is the main contributor to this harsh ailment as wells as other cardiovascular diseases. Meditation calms the mind and melts the stress layers blocking your mind. As you let go of all the negative thoughts in your mind you lower your stress hormones and as a consequence reduce heightened blood pressure.

Blood pressure, when at the optimum scale results in better sleeping & eating patterns, greater control over emotions and an overall satiated life.

# Chapter #11: Pain Relief

No one likes pain that just shows up out of nowhere. No doubt that pain plays a vital role in signaling us of due danger but uninvited chronic pain can ruin one's life. Most people counter pain by ingesting pain killers and other drugs without worrying about the side effects they inflict on their bodies.

Meditation is a much better and most importantly affect alternative to these drugs to counter the harmful effects of chronic pain. When you fail pain you are most likely to fight against it and this struggle only increases the intensity of pain and does no good meditation targets this ailment by taking your mind off the pain and providing you the ability to relax. Meditation does not result in farfetched results right away but after a few meditative periods a noticeable difference is felt in the amount of pain.

Thus, instead of turning to drugs you can practice meditation to immediately relieve you of pain by exerting your mind over things that matter and out of the physical state. A stronger spiritual mind set provides you tremendous control of your body and hence you feel relieved.

# Chapter # 12: Improved Digestion

Meditation can also help you with digestive problems such as cramps, gas or bloating. At this point it would be quite clear that meditation is not just for spiritual enlightenment but for physical welfare too. Digestion is one of the biological processes that are affected most by anxiety and stress. By reducing stress and anxiety, the body benefits in terms of greater circulation of oxygenated blood resulting in a greater quality of blood supply to the intestines and stomach.

By relaxing the mind, meditation takes you out of the anxiety 'zone'; this 'zone' causes a halt in major bodily functions including digestive processes. Therefore, if you are constantly stressed then this stress will take over as the primary concern of the mind and your body will not benefit in any way from this; so start meditation to bring back your body on the right track.

Still, remember that meditation is not a substitute for an unhygienic diet. It can only help you if your problems are stress related.

# Chapter # 13: Cure Headaches

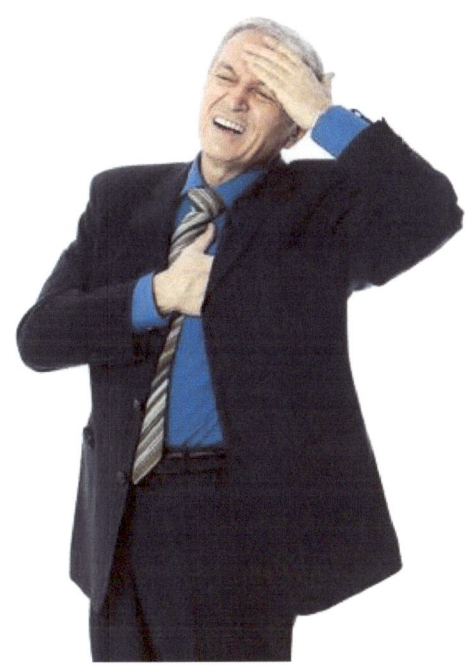

In addition to boosting immunity and curing cardiovascular ailments, meditation also reduces the intensity and with greater practice even eliminates chronic conditions such as headaches and migraines. Headaches may sound too little of a problem but those who experience it can do pretty much anything to get rid of it. This is where a free and effective solution comes in i.e. meditation.

For starters, meditation scans your body and removes every inch of tension from your body. Headaches are caused majorly bodily tensions especially those that are held in joints of the body. When you sink into your meditative technique you naturally relax your body and let go of the clenching that sits in your bones.

This hypothesis is backed up by Herbert Benson, Helen P Klemchuck and John R Graham, researchers at Harvard University. They found out that people who engaged themselves in meditation reported chronic incidents 50% less than those who did not meditate in any way.

Therefore, by letting go of the venomous tension known as stress you can get rid of chronic pains.

# Chapter # 14: Overcome Addictions

Millions of people scuffle through the dangerous habit known as addiction every single day. Many employ methods such as therapeutic sessions, drug patches and hypnosis tapes to overcome this problem but most fail miserably and resort back to full time drug abuse. If only these people knew how much they can reap from meditation…

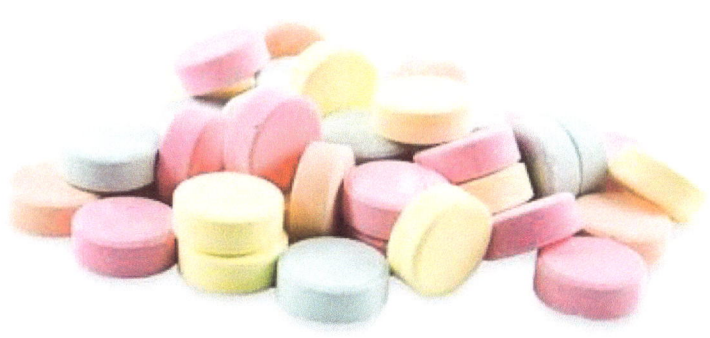

Let's come to the basics. People smoke, drink or abuse drugs to get satisfied and forget about their worries. Meditation does all these things for them and without any side effects. Meditation provides an alternative pathway to happiness and satisfaction that replaces addiction. Meditation at its core means finding inner peace, gaining serenity and letting go of fears. These benefits combine and beat the symptoms of addiction once and for all.

In addition to overcoming addictions, meditation can also help you fight unhealthy cravings and food habits. Meditation provides you greater control over your mind and body therefore; it can help you to stick to a healthy diet too.

# Chapter # 15: Lower Cholesterol Levels

What is cholesterol? It is a substance containing no calories and thus no fuel. It has various uses inside the body and in a controlled amount is necessary for the body. It is glue that holds membranes together and produces bile acids that is essential for digestion process. It also helps in the production of D vitamin and other hormones.

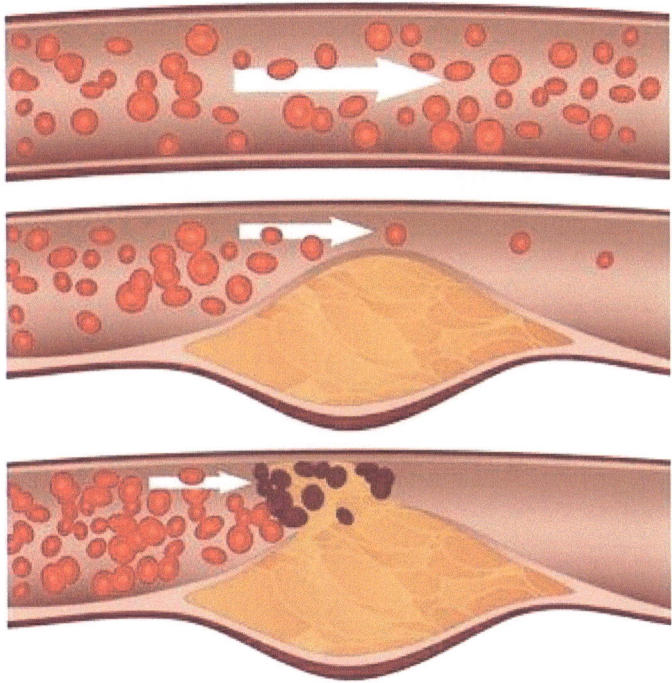

Cholesterol starts to counter act when an excess of it finds its way into the body. Cells reject this extra cholesterol and it starts to deposit in the blood vessels, clogging arteries and veins; pretty much the whole blood distribution network. When this blockade builds up in the brain, you are at the mercy of luck and can receive a stroke at any time. Furthermore, cardiovascular diseases also find their root in excess cholesterol levels.

How does meditation help? Stress causes a person to release stress hormones that act as chemicals destroying cells in the body. These broken cells need cholesterol to patch things up. Extra cholesterol finds its way through this hole and wreaks havoc in the organ. Meditation greatly counters stress and brings back the positive energy that brings stress hormone levels down. Thus, less number of cells gets damaged and therefore there is a lower chance of cholesterol getting into the body.

# Conclusion

So it is quite clear that meditation is the whole package and can improve the standard of your life greatly. From diseases ranging from headaches to heart attacks, from stress to digestive problems; meditation can provide you with the ultimate comfort and can work for you to improve the condition of your body. This book is the A-Z guide for any beginner and can teach you everything you need to know to get started into the mystic world of meditation.

So what are you waiting for? Apply what you have learnt through this book, delve into your sub-conscious and find your inner peace.

# Photo Credits

1. http://www.fotolia.com/id/51141099
2. http://www.fotolia.com/id/46908327
3. http://www.fotolia.com/id/49672671
4. http://www.fotolia.com/id/39676947
5. http://www.fotolia.com/id/51141099
6. http://www.fotolia.com/id/45156048
7. http://www.fotolia.com/id/52662791
8. http://www.fotolia.com/id/50889876
9. http://www.fotolia.com/id/45257208
10. http://www.fotolia.com/id/47136007
11. http://www.fotolia.com/id/48701190
12. http://www.fotolia.com/id/7367691
13. http://www.fotolia.com/id/27954100

# Author Bio

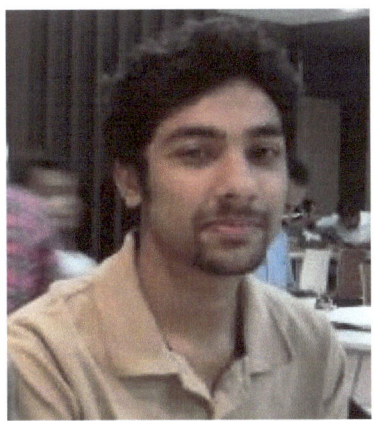

Muhammad Usman is a distinguished medical graduate of Allama iqbal medical college (AIMC). He is a professional writer who has been in the field for more than 4 years. During this time he has produced 10,000+ articles, blogs and eBooks on various niches related to diseases, health, fitness, nutrition and well-being. He is a regular contributor to several journals related to medicine and surgery. He is the editor of several journals and newspapers.

Check out some of the other JD-Biz Publishing books

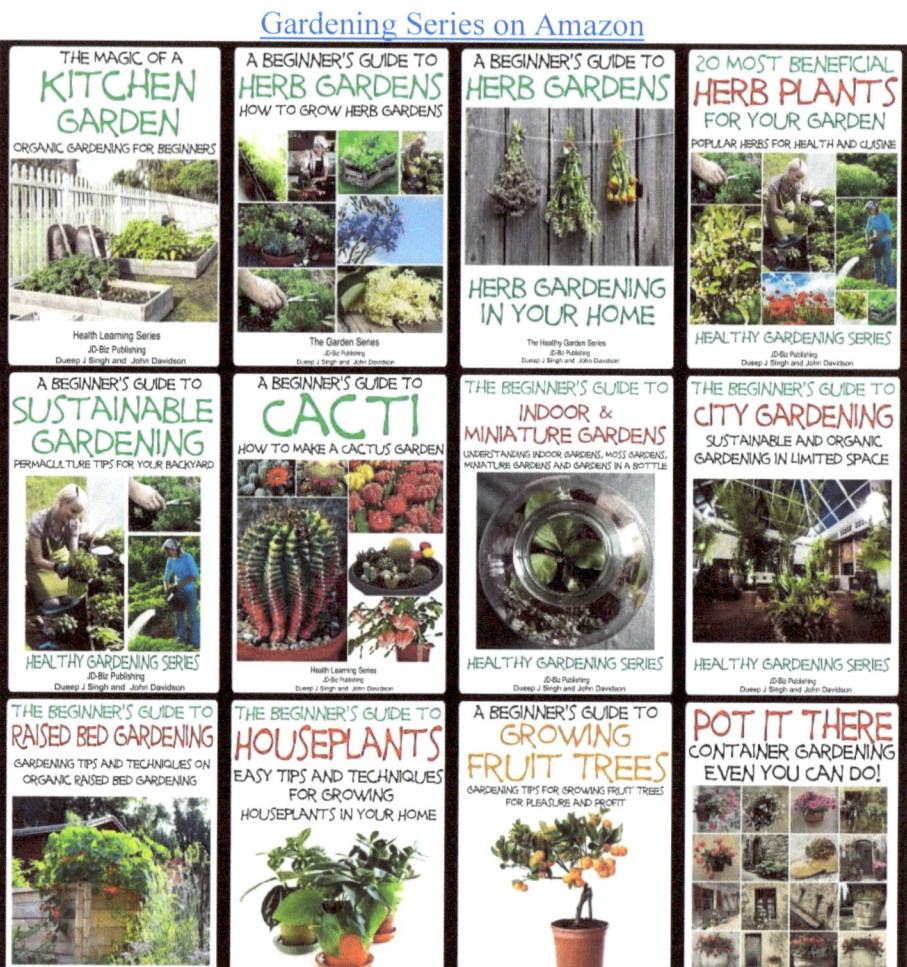

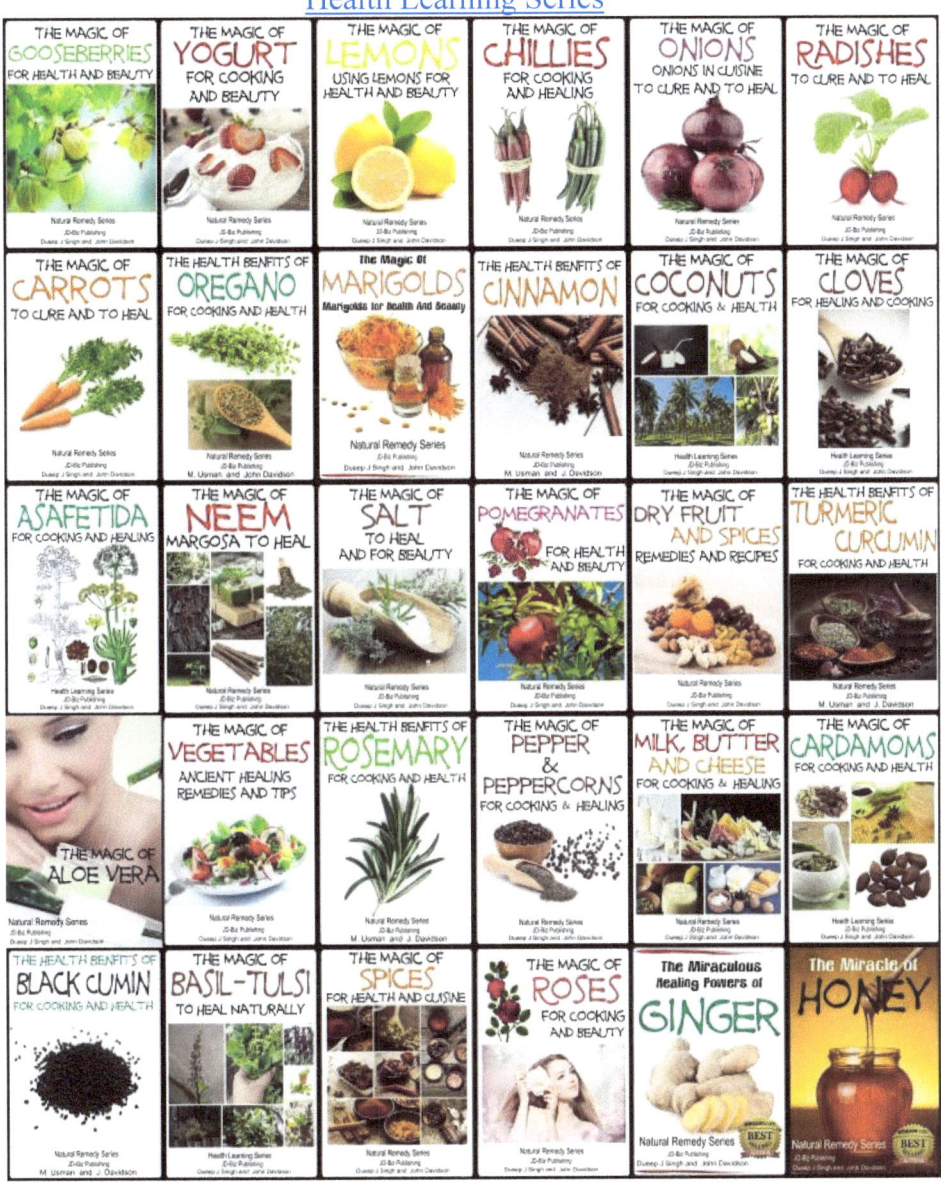

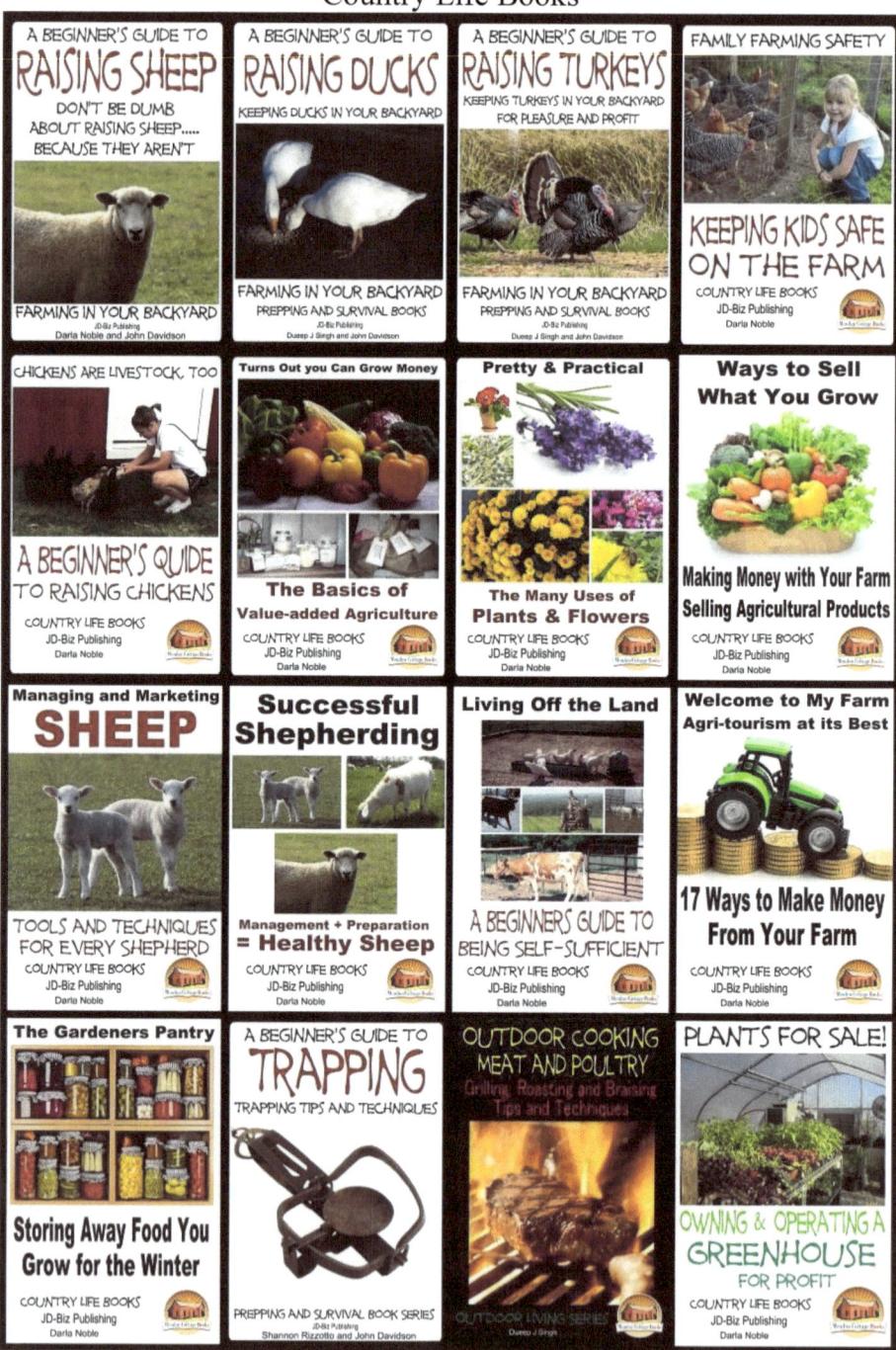

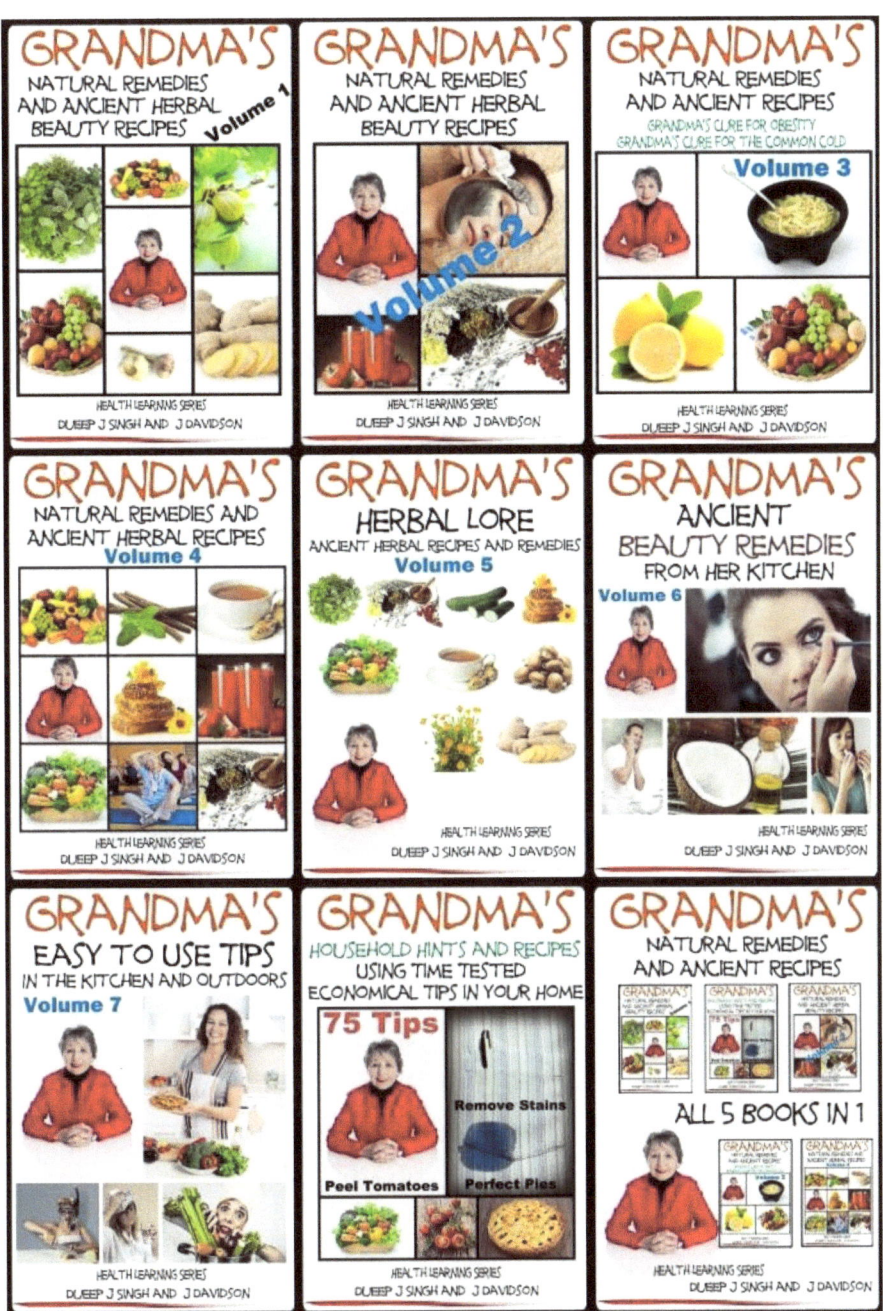

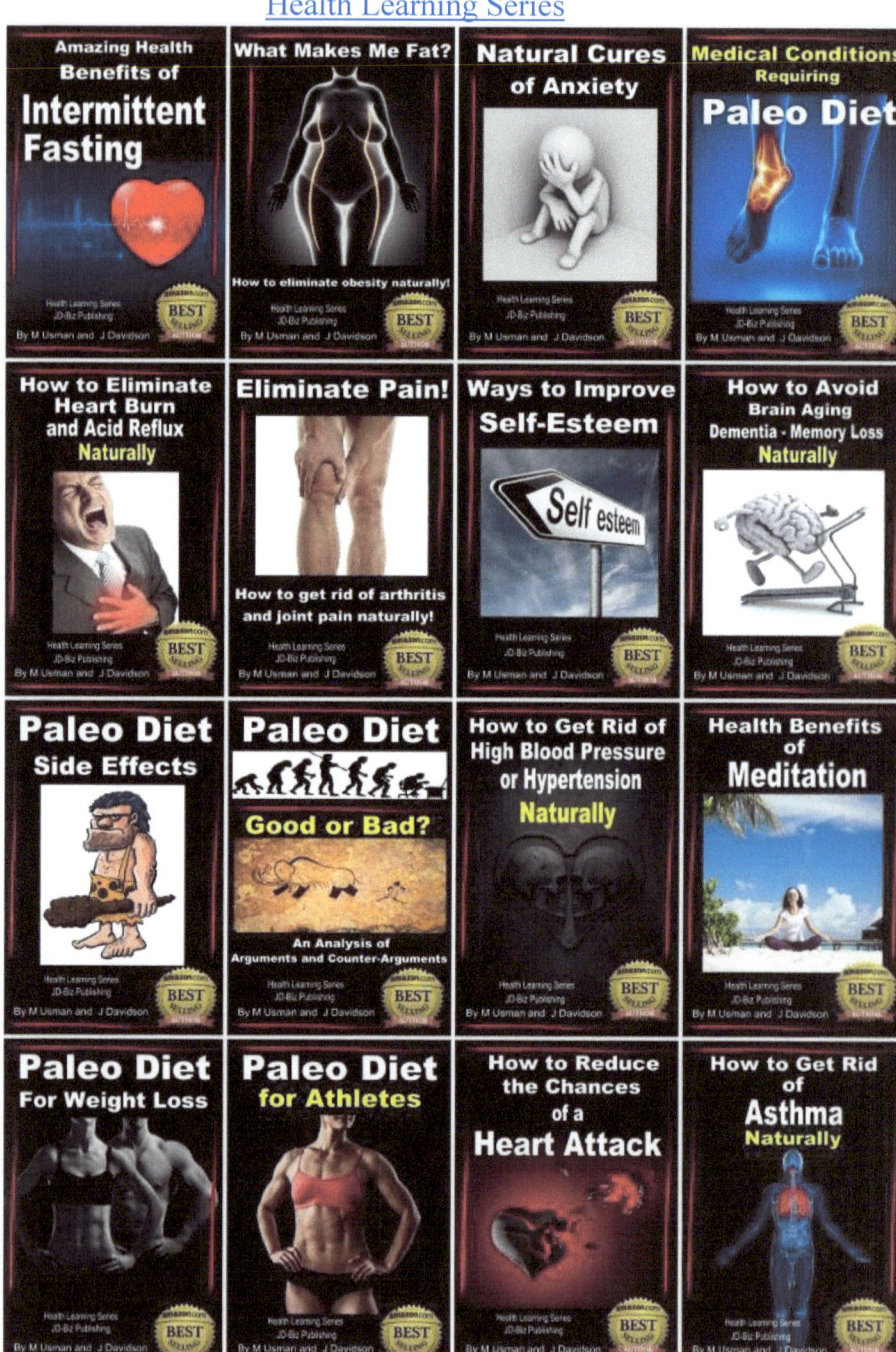

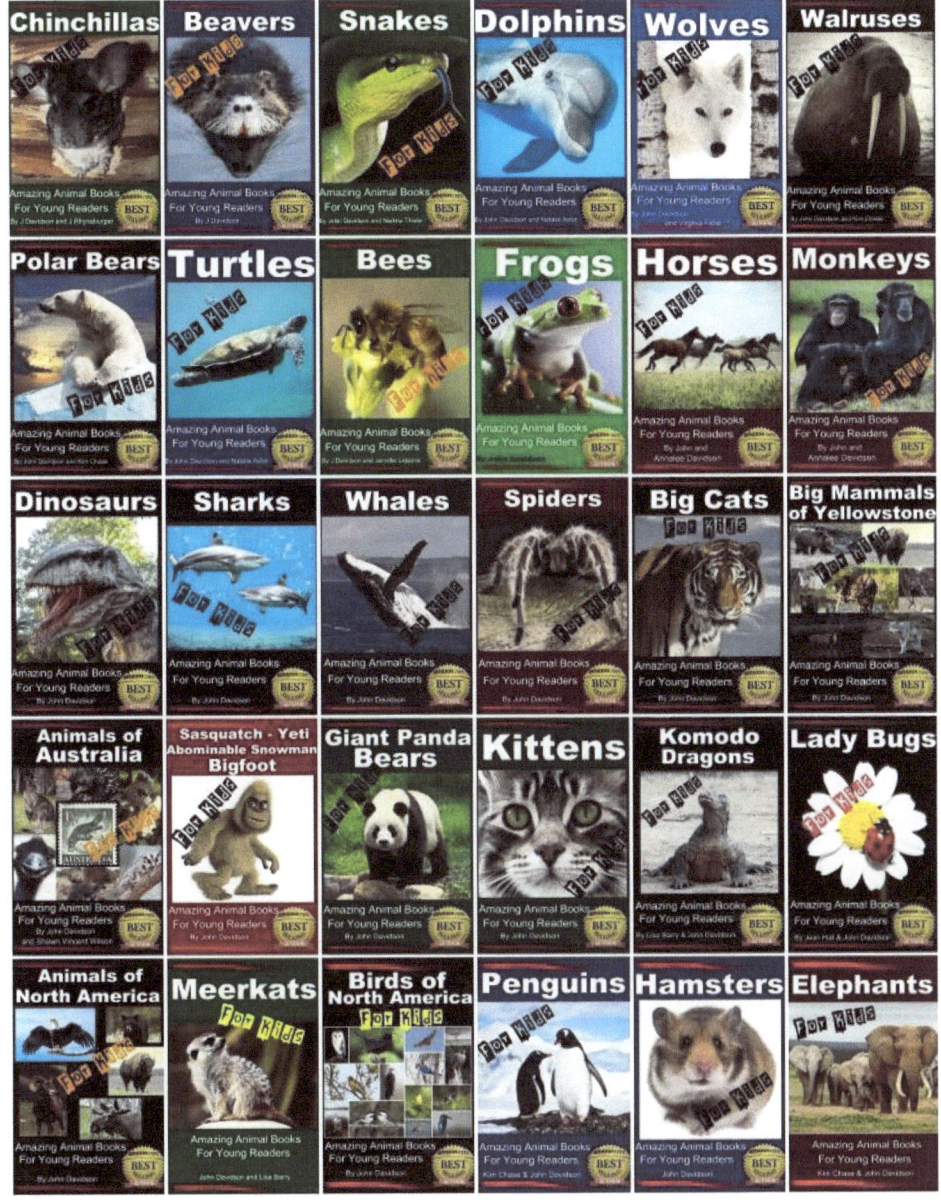

# Learn To Draw Series

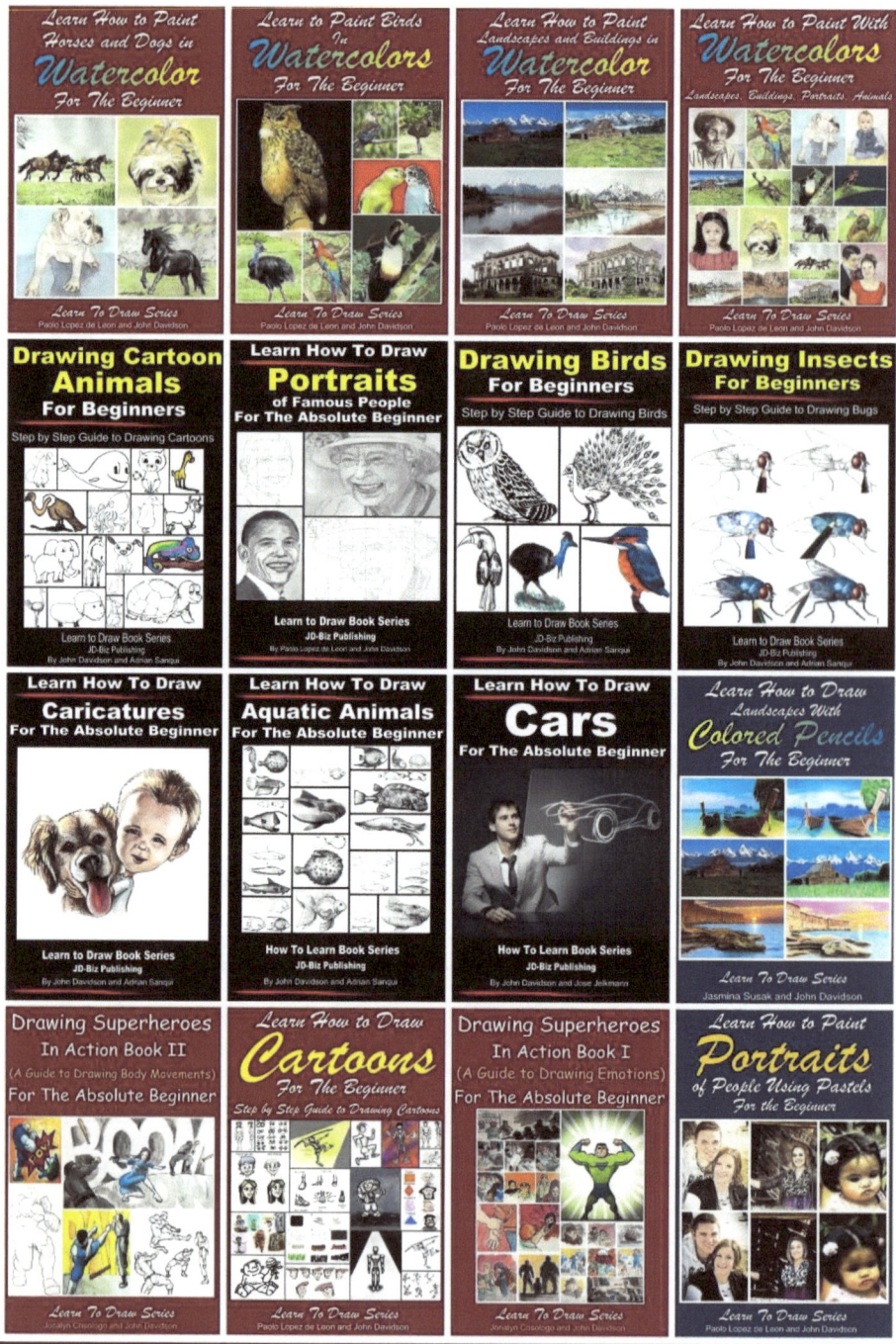

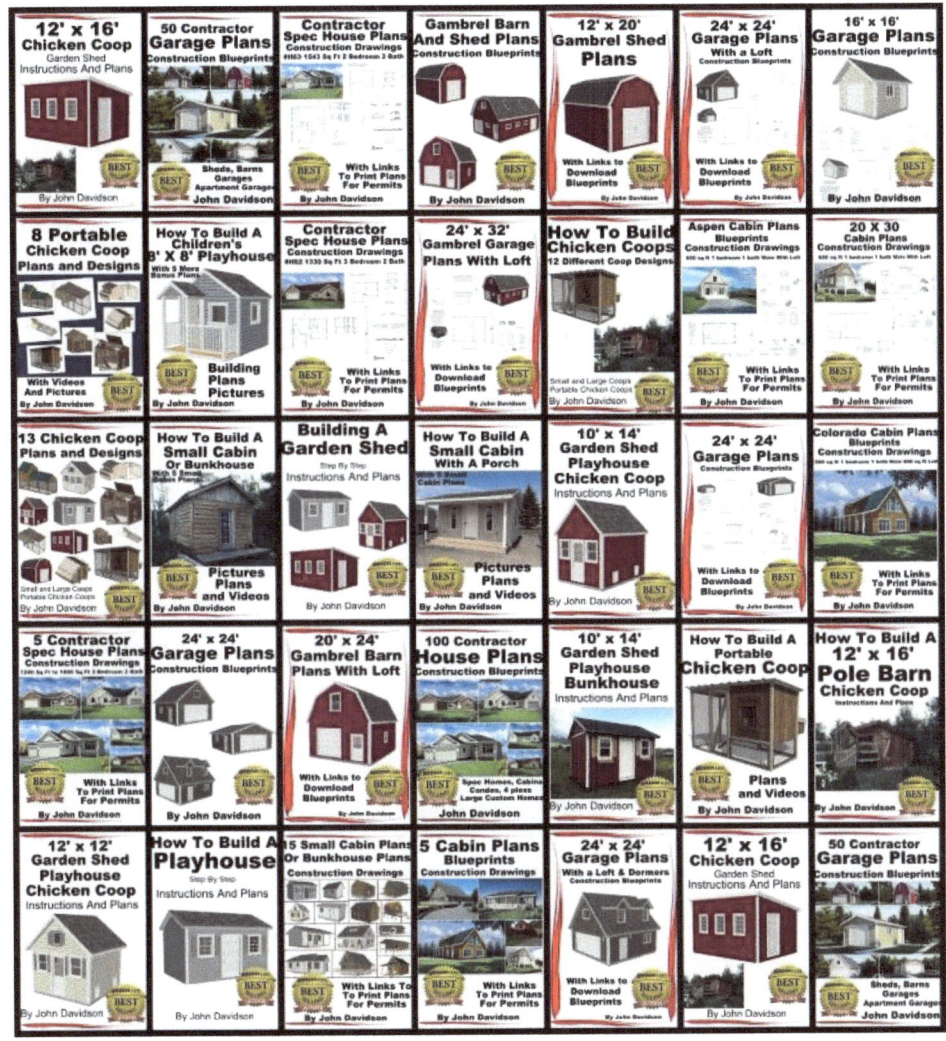

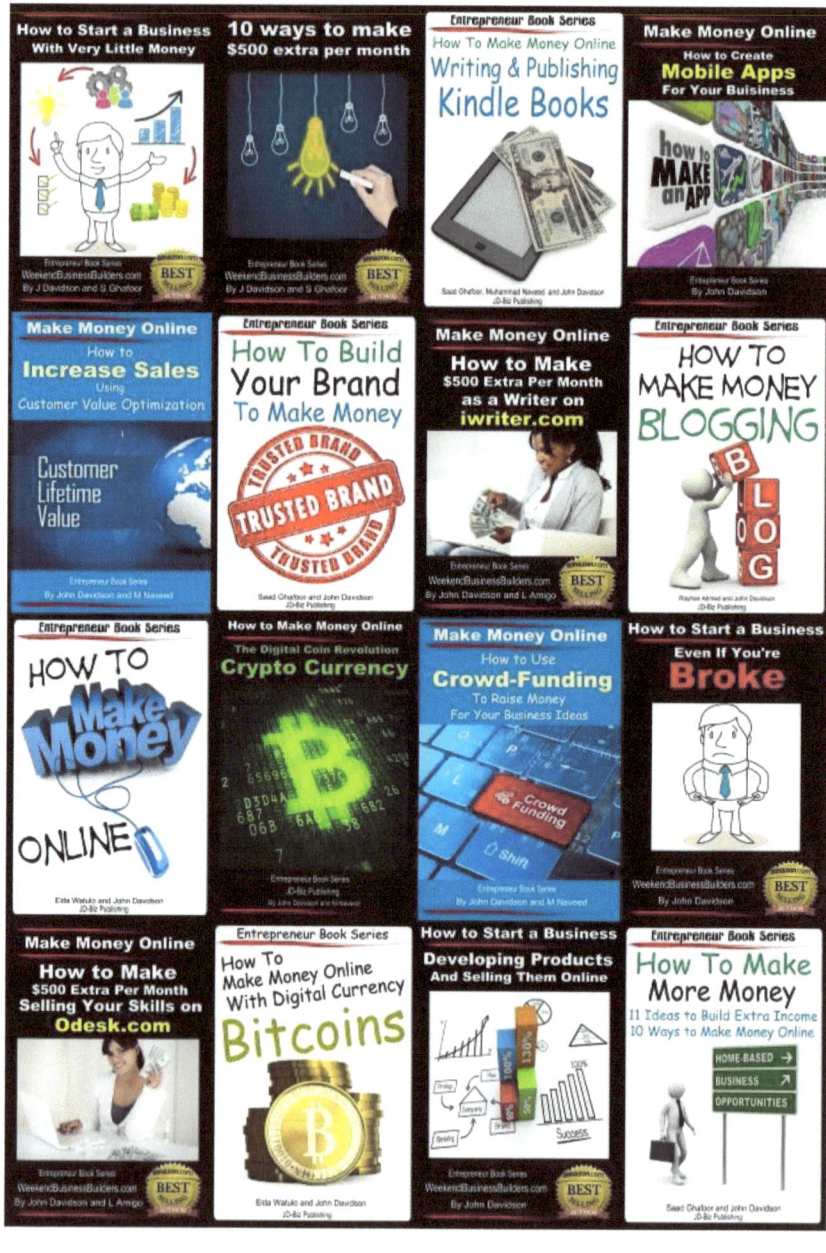

**Our books are available at**

1. Amazon.com
2. Barnes and Noble
3. Itunes
4. Kobo
5. Smashwords
6. Google Play Books


## Download Free Books!

## http://MendonCottageBooks.com

# Publisher

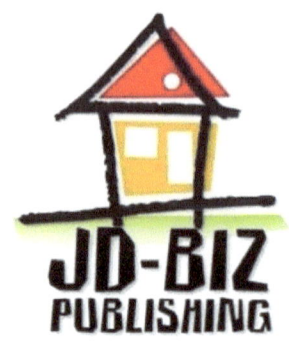

JD-Biz Corp

P O Box 374

Mendon, Utah 84325

http://www.jd-biz.com/

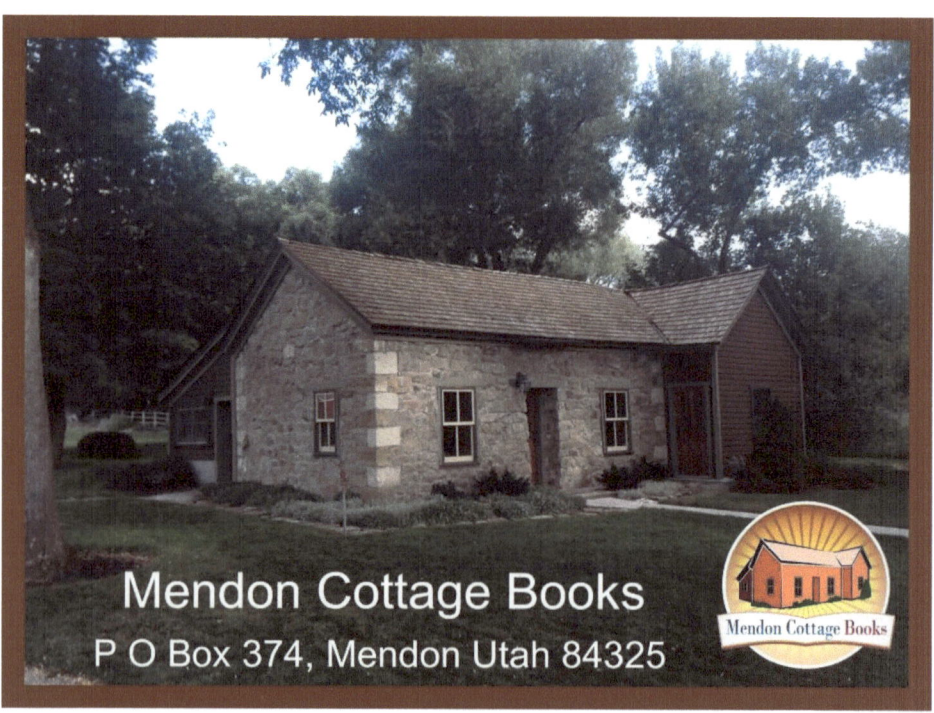

www.ingramcontent.com/pod-product-compliance
Lightning Source LLC
Chambersburg PA
CBHW050832290526
45792CB00001B/367